YOUR KNOWLEDGE HAS VALUE

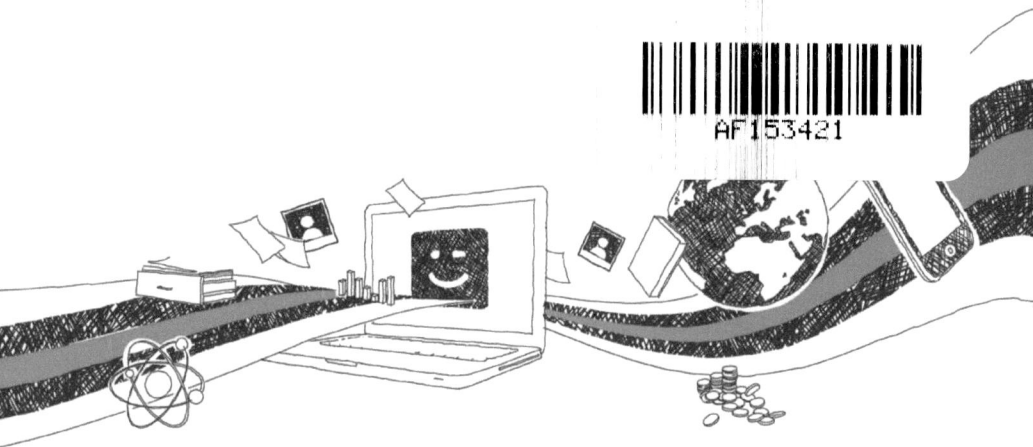
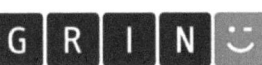

National Health Policy Thrust in Relation to Health Information Management. A Concise Review

Yusuf Popoola

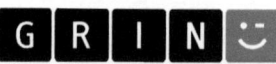

Bibliographic information published by the German National Library:

The German National Library lists this publication in the National Bibliography; detailed bibliographic data are available on the Internet at http://dnb.dnb.de.

ISBN: 9783346610300
This book is also available as an ebook.

© GRIN Publishing GmbH
Nymphenburger Straße 86
80636 München

Print and binding: Books on Demand GmbH, Norderstedt, Germany
Printed on acid-free paper from responsible sources.

The present work has been carefully prepared. Nevertheless, authors and publishers do not incur liability for the correctness of information, notes, links and advice as well as any printing errors.

GRIN web shop: https://www.grin.com/document/1184387

ABSTRACT

The National Health Policy thrust represents the collective will of the governments and people of this country to provide a comprehensive health care system that is based on primary health care. It describes the goals, structure, strategy and policy direction of the health care delivery system in Nigeria. It defines the roles and responsibilities of the three tiers of government without neglecting the non-governmental actors. Its long-term goal is to provide the entire population with adequate access not only to primary health care but also to secondary and tertiary services through a well-functioning referral system. Unfortunately, most nation states have taken "health policy" to mean "medical care policy." Medical care, however, is only one variable in a nation's health equation. The article describes what the main components of a national health policy should be, including (1) the political, economic, social, and cultural determinants of health, the most important determinants of health in any country; (2) the lifestyle determinants, which have been the most visible types of public interventions; and (3) the socializing and empowering determinants, which link the first and second components of a national health policy: the individual interventions and the collective interventions. The author discusses the indicators that should be used for each component and for each intervention. The feasibility of this approach depends to a large degree on the political will of the national authorities and the broad understanding of the actual determinants of health. A good first step is the National Health Policy plan developed by the Swedish social democratic government. This article builds on and expands on that model.

INTRODUCTION

MAJOR THRUSTS OF NATIONAL HEALTH POLICY
THE MAJOR THRUSTS OF THE NATIONAL HEALTH POLICY RELATE TO:

- **NATIONAL HEALTH SYSTEM AND MANAGEMENT**

- **NATIONAL HEALTH CARE RESOURCES**

- **NATIONAL HEALTH INTERVENTIONS**

- **NATIONAL HEALTH INFORMATION SYSTEM**

- **PARTNERSHIPS FOR HEALTH DEVELOPMENT**

- **NATIONAL HEALTH RESEARCH**

- **NATIONAL HEALTH CARE LAWS**

- **NATIONAL HEALTH SYSTEMS AND MANAGEMENT**

(a) The goal of the national health policy shall be to establish a comprehensive health care system, based on primary health care that is promotive, protective, preventive, restorative and rehabilitative to every citizen of the country within the available resources so that individuals and communities are assured of productivity, social well-being and enjoyment of living.

(b) Guaranteed minimum health care package for all Nigerians shall be the mobilizing target. As a long-term policy and within available resources, the governments of the Federation shall provide a level of health care for all citizens to enable them to achieve socially and economically productive lives.

Health System Based On Primary Healthcare

The health system, based on primary health care, shall include as a minimum:-

- An articulated programme on information, education and communication (IEC), which should also include specific programmes on school health services;
- Promotion of food supply and proper nutrition;
- An adequate supply of safe water and basic sanitation;
- Maternal and child health care, including family planning. In this context, family planning refers to services offered to couples to educate them about family life and to encourage them to achieve their wishes with regard to: preventing unwanted pregnancies; securing desired pregnancies; spacing of pregnancies; and limiting the size of the family in the interest of the family health and socio-economic status. The methods prescribed shall be compatible with their culture and religious beliefs.
- Immunization against the major infectious diseases;
- Prevention and control of locally endemic and epidemic diseases;
- Appropriate treatment of common diseases and injuries;
- Provision of essential drugs and supplies;
- Promotion of a programme on mental health; and
- Promotion of a programme on oral health.

The health system shall:

- Reflect the economic conditions, socio-cultural and political characteristics of the communities as well as the application of the relevant results of social, biomedical, health system research and public health experience;
- Address the main problems in the communities, providing promotive, preventive, curative and rehabilitative services accordingly;

- Involve, in addition to the health sector, all related sectors and aspects of state and community development, in particular agriculture, animal husbandry, food industry, education, housing, transportation, public works, communications, water supply and sanitation and other sectors, and demand the coordinated efforts of all those sectors;
- Promote maximum community and individual self-reliance and participation in the planning, organization, operation and control of primary health care, making full use of resources of Local, State and Federal Governments as well as other available resources; and
- To this end, develop, through appropriate education and information, the ability of communities to participate.

Community Involvement

(a) Governments of the Federation shall devise appropriate mechanisms for involving the communities in the planning and implementation of services on matters affecting their health.

(b) Such mechanisms shall provide for appropriate consultations at the community level with regard to local health services on the basis of increasing self-reliance. The traditional system and community organizations (cultural and religious associations) shall be fully utilized in reaching the people.

(c) The Federal and State Ministries of Health shall consult accredited groups and associations which represent the various interests within the society, including the various professional associations.

(d) The Armed Forces and Police Barracks are usually not taken care of by the Local Government Areas where they are situated. The Ministry of Defence and Police shall therefore be responsible for the health care of the citizens living in such communities.

Levels of Care

National Health Care System shall be developed at three levels viz:

Primary Health Care

i. Primary Health Care shall provide general health services of preventive, curative, promotive and rehabilitative nature to the population as the entry point of the health care system. The provision of care at this level is largely the responsibility of Local Governments with the support of State Ministries of Health and within the overall national health policy.

ii. Noting that traditional medicine is widely used and that there is no uniform system of traditional medicine in the country but that there are wide variations with each variant being strongly bound to the local culture and beliefs, the local health authorities shall, where applicable, seek the collaboration of the traditional practitioners in promoting their health programmes such as nutrition, environmental sanitation, personal hygiene, family planning and immunizations. Traditional health practitioners shall be trained to improve their skills and to ensure their cooperation in making use of the referral system in dealing with high risk patients.

Secondary Health Care

The Secondary health care level shall provide specialized services to patients referred from the primary health care level through out-patient and in-patient services of hospitals for general medical, surgical, paediatrics, obstetrics and gynaecology patients and community health services. It shall also serve as administrative headquarters supervising health care activities of the peripheral units. Secondary health care shall be available at the district, division and zonal levels as defined by the authorities of the State. Adequate specialized supportive services such as laboratory, diagnostic, blood bank, rehabilitation, and physiotherapy shall be provided.

Tertiary Health Care

Tertiary health care, which consists of highly specialized services, shall be provided by teaching hospitals and other special hospitals which provide care for specific disease conditions or specific group of patients. Care should be taken to ensure that these are evenly distributed geographically. Appropriate supporting services shall be incorporated into the development of these tertiary facilities to provide effective referral services. Selected centres shall be encouraged to develop special expertise in the advanced modern technology thereby serving as a resource for evaluating and adapting these new developments in the context of local needs and opportunities.

National Health System Management

It is generally recognized that a more effective and efficient delivery of health care can be achieved in this country by a more efficient management of the health resources. Experience has shown repeatedly that many well-conceived health schemes fail to meet expectations because of failures in implementation. It is essential to establish permanent, and systematic managerial processes for health development at all levels of care. These shall include appropriate control to ensure the continuity of the managerial process from design to application.

The National Health Managerial Process

A national managerial process shall be established to include the following elements.

(a) The national health policy - comprising the goals, priorities, main directions towards priority goals, that are suited to the social needs and economic conditions in the different States and form part of national, social and economic development policies;

(b) Programming - the translation of these policies through various stages of planning at the local, state and national levels into strategies to achieve clearly stated objectives.

(c) Programmed budgeting - the allocation of health resources by Governments of the Federation for the implementation of these strategies;

(d) Plan of Action - describing strategies to be followed and the main lines of action to be taken in the health and other sectors to implement these strategies.

(e) Detailed programming - the conversion of strategies and plans of action into detailed programmes that specify objectives and targets and the technology, manpower, infrastructure, financial resources, and time required for their implementation through the health system;

(f) Implementation - the translation of detailed programmes into action so that they come into operation as integral parts of the health system; the day-to-day management of programmes and the services and institutions for delivering them, and the continuing follow-up of activities to ensure that they are proceeding as planned and scheduled;

(g) Evaluation - of health development strategies and operational programmes in order to progressively improve the effectiveness and efficiency of their implementation;

(h) Reprogramming - with a view to improving the master plan of action or some of its components, or preparing new ones as part of a continuous managerial process for national health development.

(i) Relevant health information - to support all these components at all stages to ensure regular and wide dissemination of needed information.

> ## NATIONAL HEALTH CARE RESOURCES

Background

Resources for health development are important, albeit, indispensable component for an effective and efficient health care delivery. The appropriate and targeted applications of these resources, (material and non-material) in the right mix (quality and quantity), at the right places and in time shall be central for achieving the goals and objectives of the National Health Policy.

National Health Manpower Development

Planning human resources for health shall include:

a. Revitalizing and providing appropriate and quality human resources for health care delivery at all levels

b. Ensuring equitable distribution of human resources for health care delivery between urban and rural areas including difficult terrain such as mountainous, riverine and inaccessible area in the country.

c. Promoting collaboration among human resources for health care delivery at all levels, at the tertiary and secondary levels with and among those in cognate private and public health institutions.

d. Ensuring adequate staff at all levels in line with health sector development plans.

The policy shall ensure that:

(a) Institutions for the training of traditional health practitioners are accredited by a regulatory board.

(b) The regulatory board, from time to time, reviews curricula for training of traditional health practitioners and provides appropriate guideline towards their integration into the mainstream of Health care delivery.

(c) Traditional health practitioners are to be retrained and certificated in order to increase their skills and effectiveness in line with the regulatory guidelines.

(d) Traditional health practitioners are instructed on how to make effective use of the referral system of orthodox medical care.

Monitoring and Evaluation

Monitoring and evaluation are fundamental activities aimed at ensuring the satisfactory performance of the health care delivery system. The Human Resources for Health Development unit at all levels shall be strengthened to perform their statutory functions.

The policy shall ensure:

a. that the Human Resources for Health Development unit at federal, state and local government authorities, in collaboration with other agencies, monitor and evaluate all health care institutions within their area of jurisdiction annually to ensure their compliance with human resources for health development norms, and sanctions imposed where appropriate.

b. monitoring and evaluation reports contribute significantly to personnel training, placement and reward at all levels

Financing For Human Resources for Health

In order to achieve the aims and objectives of human resources development the policy shall prescribe the following:

a. Minimum of 15% of the health allocation shall be devoted to human resources for health development.
b. Private sector participation in human resources for health development through foundations, philanthropies, and endowments shall be encouraged.

Food, Drugs and Vaccines, Dressings and Quality Control

There shall be consistent implementation of the National Drug Policy at all levels of health care delivery in view of the centrality of efficacious drugs to the success of the health care system. Steps be taken to:-

(a) Draw up a list of essential drugs and vaccines and set up mechanisms to ensure that these drugs are available and are rationally used at all levels of the health care system;
(b) Develop local capability to produce essential drugs, vaccines and dressings and to reduce the dependence on imports by offering suitable incentives to firms which are engaged in the local manufacture, research and development of drugs;
(c) Keep surveillance on the quality of food, drugs, cosmetics and other regulated products through effective monitoring of importation and distribution channels and enforcement of relevant regulation; develop a system of monitoring drugs' adverse effects;
(d) Establish efficient systems for the procurement, storage and distribution of drugs and vaccines including a reliable "cold chain" for the latter;
(e) Allocate resources for relevant drug research including traditional remedies;
(f) Control the advertisement of drugs and other health related regulated products.
(g) Establish Drug Information Centres at all levels;
(h) Establish guidelines for clinical trial of new drugs;
(i) Establish guidelines for drug donations;
(j) Allocate specific percentage of total health budget to drugs.

Equipment

(a) The selection, ordering and maintenance of equipment and devices (e.g., x-ray machines, anaesthetic equipment, refrigerators) shall be rationalized so as to obtain savings in the cost of purchase and maintenance as well as ensuring reliable service.
(b) Existing maintenance units in tertiary and secondary health facilities shall be strengthened to be more effective and efficient to facilitate enduring maintenance culture.
(c) Ministries of Health shall co-operate by exchanging information, by standardization of specifications and by the sharing of facilities for the maintenance of equipment.
(d) Technological transfer and training shall be part of contracting conditions for purchase of complex and sophisticated medical equipment

Health Care Facilities

Ministries of Health, in collaboration with relevant bodies shall review the distribution and types of existing health care facilities and their status and shall work out a master plan of minimum requirements for health centres, dispensaries and first level referral hospitals. These plans include the repair, refurnishing, up-dating and equipping of facilities in accordance with established guidelines for each type of facility. Proposals for adequate maintenance, with community support and involvement to the extent feasible, shall also be included in this master plan. The ministries shall establish mechanisms for the issuance of Certificate of Need and Standards to regulate the location and quality of health facilities.

National Health Care Financing

(a) The Federal, State and Local Governments shall review their allocation of resources to the health sector to bring them in line with internationally recommended standards. Within available resources, high priority shall be accorded to primary health care with particular reference to under-served areas and groups. Community and financial sector resources shall be mobilized in the spirit of self-help and self-reliance. The guiding principles for the development of the national health care financing strategy/policy shall be equity, availability, acceptability, accessibility, affordability and efficiency in resource use, collaboration between all levels of government, partnerships, community participation and sustainability.

(b) In the light of the importance of health in socio-economic development, all Governments of the Federation shall review their financial allocation to health in relation to the requirements of other sectors of the economy. High priority programmes for primary health care shall have the first consideration on any additional resources that may be available.

(c) Within the health care system, efforts shall be made to redistribute financial allocation among promotive, preventive and curative health care services to ensure that adequate emphasis and awareness shall be placed on promotive and preventive services without compromising curative health services.

(d) Governments of the Federation shall explore additional avenues for financing the health care system especially health insurance schemes and health development levies.

(e) As a general policy, users shall pay for curative services, but preventive services shall be subsidized. Generally, public assistance shall be provided to the socially and economically disadvantaged segments of the population.

(f) Governments of the Federation shall encourage employers of labour and their employees to participate in financing health care services through the organization and implementation of health insurance schemes.

(g) Within the rights of individuals to participate in the economy of the nation, private individuals shall be encouraged with generous tax breaks to establish and finance private health care services in under-served areas.

(h) Within the concept of self-reliance, communities shall be encouraged to finance health care directly or find local community solutions to health problems through contribution of labour and materials and the retention of public hospital fee revenue.

(i) Mechanisms shall be established to undertake continuing studies on the benefit of various health programmes in relation to the costs, as well as the effectiveness of different technologies and ways of organizing the health system in relation to the cost and revenue;

(j) The construction and institutionalisation of National Health Account shall provide information/basis for the review of the national health care financing strategy from time to time.

> ## NATIONAL HEALTH INTERVENTIONS

It is imperative that in order to attain the national goal of achieving health for all Nigerians, an attempt should be made to address disease burdens and other health problems that significantly contribute to poor health status of Nigerians. There is a need to mount appropriate health interventions capable of achieving these objectives.

Hiv/Aids

The overall goal of the HIV/AIDS Policy is to: control the spread of HIV in Nigeria; provide equitable care and support for those infected by HIV; and mitigate its impact to the point where it is no longer of public health, social and economic concern, such that all Nigerians will be able to achieve socially and economically productive lives free of the disease and its effects.

Objectives

Objectives of the policy include:

i. fostering behaviour change as the main means of controlling the epidemic;

ii. improving national understanding and acceptance of the principle that all persons must accept responsibility for prevention of HIV transmission and the provision of care and support for those infected and affected;

iii. Providing access to cost-effective care and support for those infected, including anti-retroviral drugs.

Malaria

Reduce mortality and morbidity due to malaria

Objectives

- To reduce by 50%, the present mortality and morbidity due to malaria in children under the age of five years by the end of the year 2010.
- To reduce mortality due to malaria among pregnant women by 50% by the end of the year 2010.
- To achieve a 20% reduction in malaria case fatality and its effects, mainly in pregnant women and children by the year 2010

Immunization

The main goal of the policy is to develop and promote immunization programmes geared towards reduction of childhood morbidity and mortality through adequate immunization coverage of all at risk populations.

Objectives

- To provide the framework and guidelines for the implementation of immunization schedule for the target and at risk population.
- To provide comprehensive guidelines to assure compliance with established plans to detect, control and/or eliminate the occurrence of Vaccine Preventable Diseases (VPDs)

National Blood Transfusion

Make available at all times, blood and blood products that are safe for transfusion, by instituting a system of voluntary non-remunerative blood donation.

Objectives

a. Establish and coordinate blood transfusion services on a countrywide basis within the National Health Plan.
b. Develop a system of blood donor mobilization and motivation based on a voluntary non-remunerative donation of blood.
c. Ensure the delivery of blood, blood components and blood derivatives, which are safe for transfusion and other medical therapy.
d. Ensure the equitable distribution of equipment and consumables.
e. Maintain a system of Total Quality Management (TQM) and haemovigilance at all levels of the service.
f. Provide the modalities for manpower recruitment, training and development to satisfy the needs of the service.
g. Establish a data information support system.
h. Encourage research into all aspects of blood transfusion.
i. Maintain a cost-effective service.
j. Strive to up-hold high ethical practices.

The National Drug Policy

The goals of the National Drug Policy are to make available at all times to the Nigerian populace adequate supplies of drugs which are effective, affordable, safe and of good quality; also to ensure rational use of such drugs.

Objectives

The key objectives of the National Drug Policy are: -

(i) To ensure access to safe, effective, affordable and good quality   drugs at all levels of health care on the basis of health needs;

(ii) To promote rational use of drugs;

(iii) To increase local drug manufacture and promote export;

(iv) To promote research into both pharmaceutical raw materials and   herbal remedies;

➤ NATIONAL HEALTH INFORMATION SYSTEM

The availability of accurate, timely, reliable and relevant health information is the most fundamental step toward informed public health action. Therefore, for effective management of health and health resources, governments at all levels have overriding interest in supporting and ensuring the availability of health data and information as a public good for public, private and NGOs utilization.

The planning, monitoring and evaluation of health services are hampered by the dearth of reliable data on a national scale. Until recently, the basic demographic data about the size, structure and distribution of the population were unreliable. The system for the registration of births and deaths on a national scale is not satisfactory. Also, the system of collecting basic health data on births,   deaths, the occurrence of major diseases and other health indicators on a country-wide basis is still developmental. The available estimates are obtained from some centres where such data are collected, from national surveys, from institutional records and from special studies.

Establishment of the Information System

A national health information system shall be established by Governments of the Federation. It shall be used as a management tool for informed decision making at all levels:-

(a) To assess the state of the health of the population, to identify major health problems and to set priorities on the local, state and national levels;

(b) To monitor the progress towards stated goals and targets of the health services;

(c) To provide indicators for evaluating the performance of the health services and their impact on the health status of the population;

(d) To provide information to those who need to take action, those who supplied the data and the general public.

Development of the Information System
The development of the information system shall proceed as follows:

(a) The information system shall be developed in a phased manner starting with the simplest data which can be collected at the peripheral institutions. Efforts shall be made to implement community based systems for the collection of vital health statistics of births and deaths. Such data shall be used for planning and monitoring of health services at the local level.

(b) The State Ministry of Health shall promote and support the collection of data by the Local Government Health Authorities to improve the quality and quantity of the information. The methods of collection and recording shall be standardized as far as possible to facilitate their collation and comparison.

(c) As and when feasible, State Health Authorities shall use simple electronic data processing equipment for storage, retrieval and analysis of the data.

(d) At the Federal level, in collaboration with the National Population Commission, the Federal Office of Statistics, the Statistics Branch of the Federal Ministry of Health shall be responsible for obtaining, collating, analyzing and interpreting health and related data on a national basis. The branch shall support the State Health Authorities in the development of their information systems.

(e) Data collection and reporting of epidemics.

Monitoring and Evaluation of Health Care
For a comprehensive monitoring and evaluation of health care, minimum categories of indicators shall be as follows:

(a) Health policy Indicators,

(b) Health status Indicators,

(c) Socio-economic indicators related to health and living standard,

(d) Provision and utilization of health care indicators.

Health Policy Indicators
Health policy indicators shall include:

i. political commitment for "Health for All"; especially enactment of any necessary legislation to effect the commitment;

ii. financial resources allocation in terms of the proportion of the Gross National Product spent on health; the proportion of the total governments expenditure going to health and specifically to primary health care; and per capita government expenditure on health described by States and Local Government Areas;

iii. distribution of health resources, financial, manpower, physical facilities to reflect the degree of equity by geography and by the urban/rural ratios;

iv. Degree of community involvement. Government of the Federation are to devise appropriate mechanisms for supporting and involving the communities in the planning and implementation of health services. At least one representative from women groups or association should be a member of such committee(s).

v. Organizational framework for managerial process. vi. Universal access to essential drugs and vaccines.

Health Status Indicators

Health status indicators shall include:

i. nutritional status as indicated by birth weight of babies, weight and height measurement of infants and children in relation to age:
  - Birth weight 2500 gm or above,
  - Percentage of under - 5 malnourished,

ii. infant mortality rate,

iii. child (1 - 5 years) mortality rate,

iv. maternal mortality rate,

v. crude death rate,

vi. crude birth rate,

vii. life expectancy at birth, and at 5 years of age,

viii. Total fertility rate.

ix. HIV prevalence

Social and Economic Indicators

Social and Economic Indicators shall include:

i. rate of population increase,

ii. gross national or domestic product

iii. income distribution,

iv. work conditions,

v. adult literacy rate by sex,

vi. food availability,

vii. housing condition,

viii. basic sanitation/access to safe water,

ix. School enrolment by sex.

x. integrated transport system

xi. unemployment rate

xii. poverty index

Provision and Utilization of Health Care Indicators

Provision and utilization of health care indicators shall include coverage by primary health care and referral support:-

i. information and education concerning health; proportion of population with access to mass media outlets and measurement of adult literacy activities to the community;

ii. food and nutrition;

iii. Water supply and sanitation as above;

iv. family health indicators including proportion of children receiving child health services; proportion of pregnant women receiving antenatal, post-natal care and proportion of eligible women receiving family planning advice;

v. immunization indicators shall include the percentage of children at risk who are fully immunized against the major childhood diseases; the incidence of the six diseases in the children under 5 years of age group; and mortality rate due to the six diseases in children under 5 years of age;

vi. prevention and control of epidemic and endemic diseases indicators shall specify disease specific incidence and prevalence rate; mortality for selected number of diseases; proportion of mortality rates from communicable and non-communicable diseases; eyesight and lastly vector indices;

vii. treatment of common disease and injuries indicators shall include proportion of cases of diarrhea in children under 5 years, proportion of fevers treated with antimalarial drugs, proportion of respiratory infections treated with common antibiotics, proportion of malnutrition treated with supplementary feeds and proportion of injuries or accidents treated by first-aid or simple treatment;

viii. provision of essential drugs indicators shall specify provision of essential drugs, vaccines and supplies, essential drugs list and availability and accessibility of such items;

ix. coverage by referral system indicators shall state the proportion of population in a given area with access to the services within 5 kilometres or 1 hour travel time, the proportion of referred cases who made use of the services and the availability of referral services, e.g., paediatric, obstetric, surgical, medical, etc.;

x. proportion of referred cases that received feedback (two-way referral).Particular attention shall be placed by state/local health authorities on the needs of remote and isolated communities which have special logistic problems in providing access to the referral system;

xi. promotion of school health services shall specify school health instruction, school health environment (toilet, food, hygiene), school health periodic medical examination of children and community participation (community/parents/teachers) and provision of health services (school dispensary or infirmary);

xii. Promotion of mental health indicators;

xiii. Promotion of oral health indicators.

Sources of Health Data and Information

Principal sources of health data and information shall include the following:-

(a) Population and household censuses as prepared and projected by the National Population Commission and Federal Office of Statistics; household censuses will produce data on health related services such as housing, water supply, toilet facilities, overcrowding

(b) Vital Events Register - legal registration, statistical recording and reporting of vital events such as births, deaths, marriages, divorces. These registrations of vital events are available at appropriate State authority;

(c) Routine health service data dealing with morbidity and mortality, immunization, disease treatment, out-patient attendances, admissions, etc. These data should be obtained from the records of health services in both public and private institutions;

(d) Epidemiological Surveillance data to cover immunization records, notifiable diseases, and indication of disease incidence and prevalence;

(e) Disease Registers for specific morbidity and mortality shall be kept such as for cancer, sickle disease, handicapped persons, etc.;

(f) Budgetary Allocation data to be obtained from the Federal and State Ministries of Finance, and Planning; as well as the Local Government Authority;

(g) Community Surveys shall be undertaken in collaboration with the National Population Commission, Federal Office of Statistics, University Departments and non-governmental organizations; and

(h) Sentinel surveys on HIV/AIDS

(i) Data from school health periodic medical examinations e.g. prevalence of skin disease.

(j) Data/information from special national health programmes e.g. Roll Back Malaria

(k) Essential drug programme Family Planning/Reproductive Health programmes Management Information System should be an integral part of NHMIS

(l) Other health data sources including registers of health institutions and of health personnel

Health Data Consultative Committee (HDCC)

The State Ministries of Health shall establish a Health Data consultative committee to promote inter-departmental and inter-agency cooperation and collaboration in health data related matters with due cognizance given to the statutory responsibility of Department of Planning, Research and Statistics to coordinate health data and information in the state. The HDCC shall also address other critical issues in the state health data system.

Responsibilities of Each Level on Health Information System

(a) Community Level

(b) Facility Level (both public & private)

(c) Local Level:-

The Local Government Health Authority shall be responsible for:

i. the collection, analysis, utilization and dissemination of data in its area of jurisdiction;

ii. ensuring timely forwarding/sharing of data to relevant departments, agencies and programmes operating at the LGA level;

iii. ensuring forwarding of aggregated data, signed prescribed forms, to the state level; and

iv. Ensuring immediate submission of data in epidemic disease to the Epidemiology Division of the Department of Public Health of the Federal Ministry of Health.

v. training and supervision of relevant units of the health facilities within its area of jurisdiction

(d) **State Level:**

State Ministry of Health shall be responsible for:

i. collecting and aggregating relevant health data and information from all local government areas within the state;

ii. ensuring timely forwarding/sharing of data to relevant departments, agencies and programmes operating at the state level;

iii. ensuring immediate submission of data in epidemic disease to the Epidemiology Division of the Department of Public Health of the Federal Ministry of Health.

iv. Ensuring the preparation of state health profile for decision making, dissemination and feedback; and training and supervision of state health facility and LGA officials.

(e) **National Level:**

The Federal Ministry of Health shall be responsible for:-

i. the development, introduction and maintenance of an effective national health information system;

ii. the central coordination of the health information data;

iii. collecting, processing and presenting relevant and necessary information required both for national health planning and for monitoring the utilization of resources in accordance with national priorities and objectives; and

iv. Providing technical and management support to strengthen health management information   systems at all levels.

(f) The flow and feedback paths of health information shall be from the community level to the national level.

(g) A minimum of 1.5% of the budgetary allocation to health shall be set aside as support for the development of HMIS operations by all levels of government.

> ### PARTNERSHIPS FOR HEALTH DEVELOPMENT

There are many stakeholders and interest groups in the Nigerian health sector. Government at all levels provide and finance health services. Numerous bodies of national, community based religious and professional organizations also play active roles in the sector. Similarly, health is one of the sectors that receive assistance from a large number of international agencies and non-governmental organizations. It is therefore essential for government, Federal Ministry of Health in particular, to establish and sustain coordination of the roles of all the bodies that are active in the health sector through effective partnerships and collaborations. In order to attain and sustain the desired levels of health development, partnerships and collaborations between the governments in the health sector and government establishments in other sectors as well as public/private partnerships and collaborations are of crucial importance and will be actively promoted. These partnerships and collaborations will be guided by the following factors:

i.   The publicly funded health services alone cannot provide the services required by the populace especially with regard to the provision of quality care and universal coverage;

ii. The activities of the health services alone cannot lead to the achievement of the health status objectives;

iii. The private sector, especially the non-governmental organizations (NGOs) and the community based organizations (CBOs) are more innovative in providing peripheral services and mobilizing community participation in and support for health programmes;

iv. The basis for partnerships will be mutual trust; sharing of information; joint planning, policy formulation, implementation and evaluation; as well as joint financing of programmes and activities.

Accordingly, Federal and State Ministries of Health and Local Government authorities shall undertake appropriate measures to forge necessary partnerships:

Intersectoral Collaboration and Action

Ministries of Health have an important role in stimulating and coordinating action for health with other social and economic sectors that can participate in the processes of achieving health development. These include agriculture, animal husbandry, food industry, education, women development, finance, planning, science and technology, housing, water supply, sanitation and information. Ministries of health shall approach other sectors with a view to mobilizing them to take action in specific aspects:

i.   Ministries of Planning and Finance shall be approached, as appropriate, with a view to ensuring that health is accorded centrality in developmental planning and health programmes are granted adequate funding;

ii. The agriculture, housing and public works sectors shall be approached with respect to guaranteeing food security, appropriate balance between the production of food crops and cash crops; and the provision of safe drinking water and sanitation;

iii. The education sector shall be requested to participate in wide-ranging health educational activities such as curriculum development and teaching and propagation of health education subjects and issues;

iv. Those sectors responsible for public works, information and communication shall be requested to facilitate the provision of primary health care and to enhance the people's access to health services and information;

v. The industrial sector shall be made aware of the measures required to protect the environment from pollution and to prevent occupational diseases and injuries; they will be encouraged to facilitate the implementation of such measures;

vi. The industrial sector shall also be encouraged to consider the possibility of establishing industries for the production of essential foods and drugs;

vii. The science and technology shall be encourage to give scientific and technological support in the realization of health goals.

> ## NATIONAL HEALTH RESEARCH

Priorities for health service and biomedical research shall be set and reviewed in collaboration with the Federal Ministry of Education and the Federal Ministry of Science and Technology and the Federal Ministry of Justice. Mechanisms shall be devised to promote support and co-ordinate research activities in the high-priority areas and to strengthen the research capabilities of national institutions to enable them to undertake these essential tasks. The objectives of the health research policy are:

i. Establish the criteria for identifying priorities;

ii. Provide the operational guidelines for health research (ethical, institutional, social, legal, monitoring and evaluation etc.);

iii. Provide the framework for the coordination of health research;

iv. Identify the roles and functions of various actors and institutions and empower them;

v. Establish a sustainable mechanism for capacity development and enhancement of health research;

vi. Establish the mechanism for funding;

vii. Build consensus on health research outcomes through advocacy; viii. Disseminate information on health research outcomes widely; and ix. Promote the use of health research outcomes in addressing major health issues and problems.

Research Activities

In collaboration with the Federal Ministry of Education and the Federal Ministry of Science and Technology, Federal Ministry of Justice, the Ministry of Health and other related Ministries shall set and review:

(a) The priorities for health services and biomedical research in Nigeria. Particular attention will be paid to practical, problem solving activities including the assessment of health technologies that are being selected for use in the health services;

(b) The scope, location, capacity and content of activities in the field of biomedical and health services research at academic and other institutions;

(c) Mechanisms for promoting and financing research activities that are judged to be of high priority, and of coordinating the activities of the various scientists, researchers and institutions involved;

(d) The training of research scientists, technicians and other support staff especially in the priority disciplines where there are marked shortages, e.g., epidemiology, medical biologists, Health Care Law specialists etc.

(e) The strengthening of Ministries of Health and other institutions to enhance their capabilities to undertake relevant research.

(f) The establishment and sustainability of an outreach programme that will encourage private sector participation in health research activities.

(g) Government shall provide more resources including tax exemptions and rebates for research in the health sector and encourage the private sector, especially companies that engage in health related activities to evolve and sustain research activities that enhance health.

Biomedical and health services research shall cover the following areas:-

(i) Epidemiological research: to identify the major health problems and their determinants in different parts of the country and in different segments of the population; to incorporate the social impact assessment and the acceptability of certain treatments into research.

(ii) Operational research: to test the efficacy of health technologies and various methods of applying them in the local situation subject to the observance of medical ethics.

(iii) Developmental Research: to develop new and improved tools for the prevention, treatment and control of diseases of local importance. This will include traditional medical practices so that useful ones can be incorporated into the health care system and the practitioners can be persuaded to abandon the use of any agents or procedures (including traditional surgical operations) which are shown to be unacceptably dangerous.

(iv) Basic biomedical research: to broaden fundamental knowledge of the biological and other sciences and fields relevant to health, such as forensic medicine, medical jurisprudence and medical ethics

(v) Research on Socio-Cultural Factors Affecting Health: to identify determinants of gender issues, domestic violence, disaster/conflict management, migration/displaced people, poverty alleviation, social security system for underprivileged and disabled; and to monitor the impact and efficacy of IEC material.

Research Data Bank

In order to ensure that the priority problems in health shall be identified and addressed, and that the research results shall be adopted and applied, the Ministries of Health shall be closely involved in the planning, execution and evaluation of the research activities. The Ministries of Health shall provide a research data bank and library for the storage of research results and seek to have a law that makes it mandatory to deposit a copy with the Ministry of Health, of all health related Research Projects, Reports and These, including those leading to the award of any academic certificate or degree carried out in any Nigerian University.

Quality Assurance for Research

As a component of the health research policy, there is need for the establishment of a Good Laboratory Practice (GLP) monitoring programme in the Ministry of Health to:

a. Assure that the data received from research laboratories can be relied upon when making assessment of hazards or risks to man, animal and /or environment.

b. Examine procedures and practices used by test facilities to carry out studies and evaluate the integrity of data and the re-constructability of studies

> **NATIONAL HEALTH CARE LAWS**

One of the major weaknesses in the health sector currently is the non-existence of some important health legislations and the outdatedness, contradictions and ambiguities of some existing health laws. For example, the 1999 Constitution fell short of specifying what roles the various levels of government must play in the national health care delivery system. Therefore, one of the important health legislations that need to be put in place is the National Health Act which shall define the national health system and spell out the health actions of each level of government, among other things. Indeed, such an Act is necessary in order to give legal backing to this revised policy.

Policy Objective

To review and develop relevant legal instruments that govern and regulate health and health-related activities in the country in order to ensure that the principles and objectives of this policy are attained.

Policy Thrust

Update, formulate and disseminate laws, regulations and enforcement mechanisms related to the following:

- the development and management of the national health system (National Health Act);
- the registration and regulation of the activities of health professionals (e.g. medical and dental practitioners, pharmacists, medical laboratory scientists, public analysts, nurses and midwives, community health practitioners, chartered chemists, radiographers, optometrists and dispensing opticians, medical rehabilitation therapists, health records officers, dental technologists, traditional practitioners and other health professionals);
- the registration, manufacture, importation, storage, sale, distribution and dispensing of pharmaceuticals, vaccines, equipment and appliances, and other medical supplies;
- the general provisions for the management of the various parastatals, e.g., National Immunization Programme, National Agency for Food and Drugs Administration and Control, National Primary Health Care Development Agency, University Teaching Hospitals, Psychiatric Hospitals Management Board, Orthopaedic Hospitals Management Board, Federal Medical Centres, National Medical College, National Post-graduate Medical College of Nigeria and National Eye Hospital;
- the control of public advertising with negative impact on health and health care;
- stigmatisation and denial due to ill-health or incapacity;
- other relevant legislations

REFERENCE

- Nigeria-Revised-National-Health-Policy-2004
- https://pubmed.ncbi.nlm.nih.gov by V Navarro · 2007
- *https://vikaspedia.in › nrhm › national-health-policies*
- https://www.nhis.gov.ng
- *https://www.health.gov.ng › doc › NHPP_2019*
- *https://en.wikipedia.org › wiki › Health_policy*
- *https://pubmed.ncbi.nlm.nih.gov/17436983*

YOUR KNOWLEDGE HAS VALUE

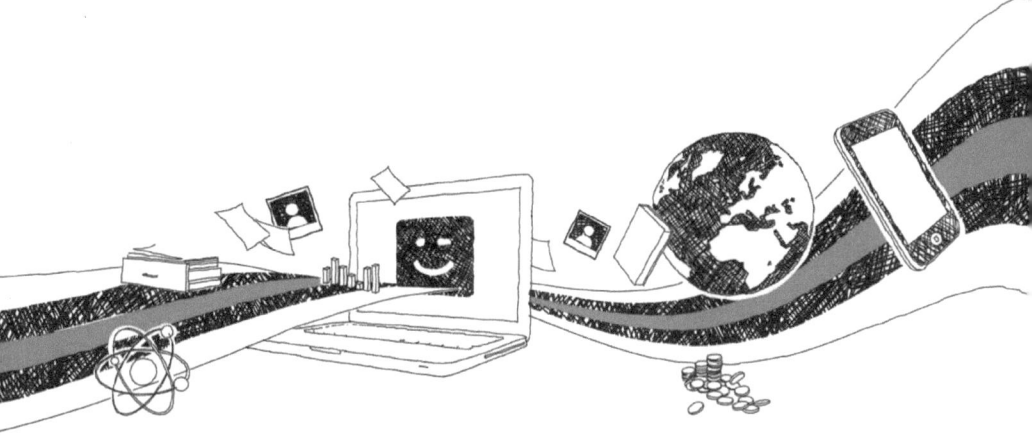

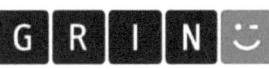